REGIMEN SANITATIS SALERNITANUM

LILIUM MEDICINAE

First Edition 12th Century

First English Edition 1608
John Harington

New Edition 2018
Edited by Tarl Warwick

COPYRIGHT AND DISCLAIMER

FOREWORD

This little work is perhaps the first comprehensive guide to diet and living. Presumably written in the 12th century (although perhaps even older) it gives a complex series of suggestions for eating, bloodletting, and treating certain ailments endemic to the Medieval period.

While the herbal and dietary material contained here is outmoded today (and while a few of its suggestions, such as ingesting orpiment, are specifically dangerous and should never be done), it does touch on certain herbal practices especially which could be seen as predominantly beneficial to those practicing it. The most easily noted example of this facet of the text is the use of willow bark, although strangely, relieving headaches is not mentioned in the same context.

We see also here a primitive explanation for modern sanitation theory; that the air lived around should be free of foul smells, specifically those of a sewer system- the miasmatic theory reigning at the time suggested that foul smells caused sickness directly- of course, living near such areas probably did overlap quite severely with epidemic sickness, due to the prevailing populations of rodents and their attendant fleas, as well as excrement, in such areas at the time.

It should be noted that within this specific edition, I have changed very little of the language, the translation from Latin already having been well completed centuries ago. I have, however, taken the liberty of reducing it from its original poetic format to fully prose, because the poetic content is no longer poetic anyways if not in the Latin which the manuscript was originally written in.

The conceptualization of the four humors, and the benefits of purging, are quite key here; indeed, about a fifth of the text deals solely with these topics. The dietary suggestions made are perhaps somewhat more interesting; any Medieval individual taking the suggestions of this text seriously would have likely been well nourished indeed, for it applauds the benefits of marrow (which is nutrient dense) along with certain vegetables notable for their vitamin and fiber content. Add to this the intake of alcohol being as high as it probably was regardless of a person's awareness of this guide, and any water drunk wouldn't have needed to be clean of parasites or harmful bacteria, for both would have been destroyed when it was mixed with the only good thing they possessed to destroy life forms they could not even see.

REGIMEN SANITATIS

If you want to be healthy, if you want to remain sound, take away your heavy cares, and refrain from anger. Be sparing of undiluted wine, eat little, get up after eating fine food, avoid afternoon naps, do not retain your urine nor tightly compress your anus. Do these things well, and you shall live a long time.

Should you need physicians, these three doctors will suffice: A joyful mind, rest and a moderate diet.

In the morning, upon rising, wash your hands and face with cold water. Move around awhile and stretch your limbs. Comb your hair and brush your teeth. These things relax your brain and other parts of your body. After your bath keep warm; stand or walk around after a meal; go slowly if you are of cool temperament.

Take a short afternoon nap, or none at all, as fever, indolence, headache and chest cold may result from that nap.

Four illnesses come from gas retained in the stomach: Spasm, dropsy, colic and vertigo.

REGIMEN SANITATIS SALERNITANUM

Your stomach will suffer great harm after a heavy meal. In order not to feel weighed down at night, make your evening meal light.

Do not eat a second time until your stomach has been purged and emptied of the food which you took earlier. You will be able to know for sure whether you are hungry, by judging your desire for food. The other sign is having dined lightly earlier.

Peaches, apples, pears, milk, cheese, salted meats, deer meat, rabbit, goat, and beef are melancholic and harmful to the sick.

Fresh eggs, red wines and rich gravies are recommended since they are nutritious in nature.

Wheat, milk, and fresh cheese are nourishing and fattening, as are testicles, pork meat, brain, marrow, sweet wines, good tasting foods, raw eggs, ripe figs, and fresh grapes.

Wines should be tested for smell, taste, brightness, and color. If you want good wines, these five things should be tested in them: How strong, brilliant, fragrant, cool, and fresh they are.

REGIMEN SANITATIS SALERNITANUM

Most nutritious are the heavy white wines.

If too much red wine is drunk, it causes constipation and raucousness of the voice.

Garlic, nuts, rue, pears, radishes, and theriaca are antidotes for deadly poison.

The air must be pure, habitable, and bright, it should be neither contaminated nor smell of the sewer.

If you develop a hangover from drinking at night, drink again in the morning; it will be your best medicine.

The best wine engenders the best humors. If wine is dark, it renders your body indolent; wine should be clear, aged, subtle, ripe, well diluted, zesty, and taken in moderation.

Beer should not be sour but clear. It should be brewed from healthy grains, and sufficiently fermented and aged.

Your stomach will not weighed down from drinking beer.

Take a moderate quantity of food in the springtime.

Summer's heat is also harmful to those who eat immoderately. In autumn beware that fruits do not become cause for mourning. Eat as much as you like in winter.

Sage and rue will make your drinks safe. If you add the flower of the rose, it will strongly diminish your lust.

Seasickness will not trouble a man who has taken seawater mixed with wine before the trip.

From sage, salt with wine, pepper, garlic, and parsley make a sauce, mixing it together in a sprightly manner.

If you want to be healthy, wash your hands often. Washing after a meal gives you two benefits: It cleans your hands and makes your eyes keen.

Bread should be neither warm nor stale. It should be leavened, raised, well-baked, moderately salted, and chosen from the best grains. Do not eat the crust, since it causes burning choler. Bread that is salted, leavened, well-baked, pure, and healthy should be of great benefit to you.

If you eat pork without wine, it is worse than mutton. If you add wine to pork, then it is food and medicine. The intestines of pigs are good; those of other animals are bad.

Must interferes with urination and acts as a laxative. It causes stoppage of the liver and spleen, and engenders kidney stones.

Drinking and eating at the same time may be harmful, since water cools the stomach, and the food is liable to remain undigested.

Veal is very nourishing.

Chicken, duck, turtledove, starling, pigeon, quail, blackbird, pheasant, thrush, partridge, chaffinch, orex, wagtail, and water fowl are nourishing.

If fish are soft, they should be eaten when they are large in size; if fish are hard, they are more nutritive when small in size.

Pike, perch, sole, whiting, tench, shrimp, plaice, carp, gurnard, and trout are all edible fish.

Eating eels is bad for the voice as those who know anything about medicine will attest, and cheese and eel are harmful when eaten together in great quantity, unless you drink wine often.

During the meal take small drinks often. If you eat an egg, make it soft and fresh.

We decided both to praise and to reproach the pea: Without the pod, peas are rather good; with the pod, they cause gas and are harmful.

Goat's milk is healthy for consumptives, and next after that camel's milk, but most nutritious of all is ass's milk; cow's milk is also nutritious and likewise sheep's milk. If your head is feverish or aches, milk is not very healthy.

Butter softens; it is moist and acts as a laxative when there is no fever.

Whey cuts through and washes, penetrates and purifies.

Cheese, is cold, constipating, crude, and hard, cheese and bread are good food for a man who is healthy; if a man is not healthy, then cheese without bread is good.

"Ignorant doctors say that I am harmful, nevertheless they do not know why I should do harm."

REGIMEN SANITATIS SALERNITANUM

Cheese brings help to a weak stomach. Taken after your other food, it properly ends the meal. Those who are not ignorant of medicine will attest to these things.

During the meal take small drinks often, so that you do not become ill, do not wait to drink in between courses.

After each egg drink another cup of wine; after fish have nuts, after meat serve cheese. One kind of nut is good, a second is harmful, a third kind brings death.

Add a drink of wine to your pear, and the nut is medicine against poison. A pear tree produces our pears. Without wine its pears are poison; if pears are poison, then damned be the pear tree!

If you cook them, pears are an antidote, but uncooked they are a poison. Raw they aggravate the stomach; cooked, pears relieve the aggravation. After the pear, drink wine; after the apple empty your bowels.

From eating the cherry, you will derive great benefits: It purges the stomach, its pit removes your kidney stone, and from its pulp will come good blood.

Plums are quite beneficial to you: they are cooling and cathartic.

REGIMEN SANITATIS SALERNITANUM

You should take peaches with must, just as it is customary to eat grapes with nuts. Raisins are bad for the spleen, but good for a cough or for the kidneys.

Fig in a poultice removes scrofula, tumor, and glandulas; add poppy and it mends together broken bones.

The fig generates lice and lust, but it resists anything.

Medlars cause excessive urine and constipation. Medlars are good hard, but better soft.

Must causes urine, is laxative and brings on gas.

Beer nourishes thick humors, gives strength, fattens the flesh, produces blood, provokes urine, has a laxative effect, causes gas, and has a cooling effect. Vinegar has more of a drying effect: It cools, makes a man thin, induces melancholy, decreases the number of sperm, harms those of dry humor, and dries up the nerve of the fats.

The turnip helps the stomach, produces gas, Causes urine, and may do harm to the teeth. If it is served under-cooked, it may give you a stomach cramp.

The heart of all animals is slow to digest and hard to

excrete. Similarly the stomach is harder to digest and excrete than its extremities.

Tongue gives good medicinal nourishment. The lung is easily digested and is quickly expelled. The brain of chickens is better than any other animals.

The fennel seed loosens gas.
Anise improves vision and comforts the stomach. And sweet anise works better.

The ashes of certain vegetable matters stop hemorrhage.

The salt dish should be placed on the table at mealtime. Salt wards off poison, and adds taste to a man's food, for food which is served without salt does not taste good. Very salty foods hurt the eyes, decrease sperm, and engenders scabies, pruritus, or vigor.

These three flavors have a warming effect: the salty, the bitter, and the sharp. The sour, like the styptic, and the acidulous have a cooling effect. The unctuous, the tasteless, and the sweet yield a balanced effect.

Wine soup has a quadruple effect: it cleans the teeth; it gives sharp vision; what is lacking it supplies; what is overabundant it reduces.

I prescribe a regular diet for all people: I recommend keeping that diet unless it is necessary to change it. Hippocrates attests that disease may result otherwise. A proper diet is one of the foremost goals of medicine; attend to your diet, or you foolishly direct your other efforts and take care of yourself badly.

What kind? what? when? how much? how often? where to be given? These things a doctor should quickly take note of while prescribing a diet.

Cabbage broth has a laxative effect; its substance is astringent; when taken together they act as a laxative.

The Ancients called mallow "malva" because it softens the belly. The roots of the mallow act as a laxative; they bring movement to the womb and cause menstrual flow to occur often.

Mint would not be mint if it were slow to expel dangerous intestinal worms of the belly and stomach.

Why should a man die in whose garden grows sage? Against the power of death there is not medicine in our gardens, but sage calms the nerves, takes away hand tremors, and helps cure fever. Sage, castor bean, lavender, primrose, nasturtium, and athanasia cure paralytic parts of the body. Oh sage the savior, of nature the conciliator!

Noble is rue since it gives you keen eyesight. With its help, certainly as a man, you will see sharply. Rue decreases coitus in man and increases it in women. Rue makes man chaste, intelligent and cunning. When cooked, rue makes the house safe from fleas.

The doctors do not seem to agree on onions. Galen says that they are not good for those of choleric humor, but he teaches that they are quite salubrious for phlegmatics, and especially good for the stomach and the complexion. By frequently rubbing your bald spots with ground onions, you may restore your head of hair.

The mustard seed is small, dry, and hot. It causes tears, relieves the head, and expels a poison.

Drunkenness and headache are relieved by the violet. They say that it also cures epileptics.

The nettle gives sleep to the sick, stops vomiting, relieves chronic cough, and is a remedy against colic. It takes away your chest cold as well as abdominal tumors, and it helps in all diseases of the joints.

REGIMEN SANITATIS SALERNITANUM

The hyssop is an herb that purges your chest of phlegm. When it is cooked with honey it is good for the lungs. It is said to restore a healthy coloring to your face.

Chervil ground and mixed with honey is a remedy for the canker. When it is taken with wine it cuts off pain; it often stops vomiting and loose bowls.

Fleabane taken with wine expels black bile; they say it also cures chronic gout.

The mother swallow uses celandine in restoring sight to her blinded young whose eyes have been plucked out, according to Pliny.

The willow's juice kills worms when poured into their ears; its bark cooked in vinegar cures warts; the juice of the fruits and the flower are harmful to human reproduction.

The saffron, being cheery, is said to comfort; it aids weak parts of the body and helps the liver.

Phlegm makes man weak, stout, short, and fat, while the blood humor makes men of medium build. Men of phlegmatic humor tend toward leisure rather than work, and dullness of senses, slow movement, laziness, and sleep are typical. Those sleepy and sluggish men, who spit often, are dull of senses and white in coloring.

If eaten often, leeks make girls fertile. You may also stop nosebleed with them.

Because pepper is black, it is not slow to dissolve. It will purge phlegm and help digestion. White pepper is good for your stomach and useful for the pain of cough. It will ward off the attack of fever and its rigor.

Both sleep and too much movement soon after eating, as well as drunkenness, are usually bad for the hearing.

Fear, long fasting, vomiting, a blow, a fall, drunkenness, and cold cause a ringing in your ear.

Baths, wines, Venus, wind, pepper, garlic, smoke, leeks, onions, lentil, weeping, beans, mustard, the sun, coitus, fire, work, a blow, spicy foods, dust: These things hurt the eyes, but staying up late hurts them more so.

Fennel, verbena, the rose, celandine, rue: From these mix juices to sharpen your eyesight.

Likewise take care of your teeth: gather the seeds of

the leeks, burn them with the juice of the henbane, and direct the smoke toward your teeth through a funnel. Nuts, olive oil, head cold, eels, drinking, and raw apples make a man hoarse.

Fast, stay awake, eat hot food, work hard, breathe warm air, drink little, hold your breath: Do these things well if you want to get rid of a cold.

If the cold goes down to the chest it is called catarrh. When it goes to the fauces, hoarseness; to the nose, coryza.

Mix sulfur with orpiment. And add quick lime, then combine them with soap. Mix these four together, and when they are mixed your fistula will be cured, when these four steps are completed.

Man has two hundred and nineteen bones. He has thirty-two teeth, and three hundred and sixty-five veins.

Elecampane is good for the diaphragm. If its juice is mixed with that of rue, there is nothing more healthful for those with hernia.

Nasturtium juice spread over the head is said to stop hair from falling out; it also cures toothache; and the juice mixed with honey cures scales.

Four humors make up the human body: Blood, choler, phlegm and melancholy. Earth corresponds to melancholy, water to phlegm, air to blood, fire to choler.

Fat and jolly of nature are those of sanguine humor. They always want to hear rumors, Venus and Bacchus delight them, as well as good food and laughter. They are joyful and desirous of speaking kind words.

These people are skillful for all subjects and quite apt. For whatever cause, anger cannot lightly rouse them. They are generous, loving, joyful, merry, of ruddy complexion. Singing, solidly lean, rather daring, and friendly.

Next is the choleric humor, which is known to be impulsive: This kind of man desires to surpass all others. On the one hand he learns easily, he eats much and grows quickly. On the other hand, he is magnanimous, generous, a great enthusiast. He is hairy, deceitful, irritable, lavish, bold, astute, slender, of dry nature, and of yellowish complexion.

There remains the sad substance of the black melancholic temperament, which makes men wicked, gloomy, and taciturn. These men are given to studies, and little sleep. They work persistently toward a goal; they are insecure. They are envious, sad, avaricious, tight-fisted, capable of deceit, timid, and of muddy complexion.

These are the humors which give to each his skin coloring:

From phlegm comes a fair, white complexion.

From blood a ruby color, and a rather tawny complexion from red choler.

If blood is overabundant, the face turns red, the eyes protrudes, the cheeks swell up, the body is too weighed down, the pulse is frequent, full, and soft; great pain occurs, especially in the forehead; the bowels are constipated. A dry tongue and thirst result, and dreams are completely red in color. The saliva is sweet, even when tasting bitter things.

Phlebotomy is scarcely needed before a person is seventeen. The more productive spirit will escape with your blood during phlebotomy, but these spirits will soon be replaced by drinking wine, and any harm done by the humors will be gradually repaired by food.

REGIMEN SANITATIS SALERNITANUM

Phlebotomy clears your eyes, freshens your mind and brain, makes your marrow warm, purges your bowels and restrains your stomach and belly from vomiting or menstruation; it purifies the senses, brings on sleep, takes away weariness; it cultivates and improves hearing, speech, and strength.

These are the good months for phlebotomy - May, September, April, which are lunar months just as are the Hydra days.

Neither on the first day of May nor the last day of September or April should blood be drawn or goose be eaten. In the old man or in the young man whose veins are full of blood, phlebotomy may be practiced in every month. These are the three months: May, September, April, in which you should draw blood in order to live a long time.

Cool constitution, a cold region, great pain, bathing, sexual intercourse, youth and old age, long illness, heavy drinking, and eating; if you are in one of these situations or if you are nauseous, then phlebotomy is not good for you.

What should you do when you want to be phlebotomized? Or when you are bloodletting or when you will have blood let? Ointment, drink, washing, bandages, and movement should be kept well in mind.

REGIMEN SANITATIS SALERNITANUM

Phlebotomy cheers the sad, calms the angry and helps cure madmen.

Make the wound rather large, so that quickly the vapors may escape, and blood come out more abundantly and more freely.

When blood has been taken out, stay awake six hours, so that the vapors of sleep will not harm your sensitive body. To avoid damaging a nerve, do not let your wound cut deep. After being cleansed by blood, you should not eat immediately.

You should avoid all milk products, and refrain from drinking after phlebotomy. Keep away from cold things, since cold is bad for you.

While in this condition, avoid walking outside during cloudy weather, but raise your spirits by walking outside in good weather. Rest is appropriate for all, and movement could prove harmful.

Practice phlebotomy at the beginning of acute and very acute illnesses. Take a lot of blood from those of middle age; from children and older persons take only a little. Take twice as much blood in spring, but only the normal amount in other seasons.

REGIMEN SANITATIS SALERNITANUM

In summer and spring take blood from the right veins; in autumn and winter from the left.

These four parts of the body- the head, the heart, the feet, the liver- should be relieved of blood.

The heart in spring, the liver in summer, the following in the order of the seasons- the head in winter, the feet in autumn.

Opening the salvatella vein gives you many small benefits: It purges the liver, the spleen, the chest, the diaphragm, and the voice; it also takes away any unnatural pain from the heart.

If your headache is from alcohol, drink water, for from too much alcohol an acute fever may occur.

If the top of your head or forehead has a burning pain, rub your temples and forehead moderately at the same time, and wash them with warm morel that has been cooked.

Fasting in summertime dries out the body. Vomiting is profitable in every month, for it purges harmful humors, and it washes the circuits of all the stomach. Spring, summer, autumn, and winter are the seasons of the year.

REGIMEN SANITATIS SALERNITANUM

In springtime the air is warm and humid, and no time is better for phlebotomy. In spring lovemaking is beneficial to man in moderation, as are exercises, laxatives, sweating, and baths. In that season the body should be purged with medicines.

Summer is usually hot, and is known as a dry season. The summer encourages the occurrences of red choler. In summer food of cold and humid qualities should be served, and lovemaking should be avoided;

Baths are not good then, and phlebotomy should be rare. Rest is useful, and drink is good in moderation.

THE END